It's easy to get lost in the cancer world

Let NCCN Guidelines for Patients® be your guide

- Step-by-step guides to the cancer care options likely to have the best results
- Based on treatment guidelines used by health care providers worldwide
- Designed to help you discuss cancer treatment with your doctors

About

National Comprehensive Cancer Network®

NCCN Guidelines for Patients® are developed by the National Comprehensive Cancer Network® (NCCN®)

NCCN

- ✓ An alliance of leading cancer centers across the United States devoted to patient care, research, and education

Cancer centers that are part of NCCN:
NCCN.org/cancercenters

NCCN Clinical Practice Guidelines in Oncology (NCCN Guidelines®)

- ✓ Developed by doctors from NCCN cancer centers using the latest research and years of experience
- ✓ For providers of cancer care all over the world
- ✓ Expert recommendations for cancer screening, diagnosis, and treatment

Free online at
NCCN.org/guidelines

NCCN Guidelines for Patients

- ✓ Present information from the NCCN Guidelines in an easy-to-learn format
- ✓ For people with cancer and those who support them
- ✓ Explain the cancer care options likely to have the best results

Free online at
NCCN.org/patientguidelines

NATIONAL COMPREHENSIVE CANCER NETWORK FOUNDATION
Guiding Treatment. Changing Lives.

and supported by funding from NCCN Foundation®

These NCCN Guidelines for Patients are based on the NCCN Guidelines® for Management of Immunotherapy-Related Toxicities (Version 1.2020, December 16, 2019).

NCCN Foundation seeks to support the millions of patients and their families affected by a cancer diagnosis by funding and distributing NCCN Guidelines for Patients. NCCN Foundation is also committed to advancing cancer treatment by funding the nation's promising doctors at the center of innovation in cancer research. For more details and the full library of patient and caregiver resources, visit NCCN.org/patients.

National Comprehensive Cancer Network (NCCN) / NCCN Foundation
3025 Chemical Road, Suite 100
Plymouth Meeting, PA 19462
215.690.0300

Endorsed by

Be the Match®

National Marrow Donor Program® (NMDP)/Be The Match® is the global leader in providing a possible cure to patients with life-threatening blood and marrow cancers, as well as other diseases. Our Be The Match Patient Support Center provides support, information, and resources for patients, caregivers, and families. BeTheMatch.org/one-on-one

Good Days

Good Days is proud to support this educational resource for patients and their families and offers unwavering commitment to those who struggle with chronic disease, cancer, and other life-altering conditions.mygooddays.org

Stupid Cancer

Stupid Cancer's mission is to empower adolescents and young adults affected by cancer by ending isolation and building community. Through our innovative programming and strategic communications platforms, our goal is to provide support, resources, education, and a sense of community through online and in-person programming. stupidcancer.org

The Leukemia & Lymphoma Society

The Leukemia & Lymphoma Society (LLS) is dedicated to developing better outcomes for blood cancer patients and their families through research, education, support and advocacy and is happy to have this comprehensive resource available to patients. lls.org/informationspecialists

To make a gift or learn more, please visit NCCNFoundation.org/donate or e-mail PatientGuidelines@nccn.org.

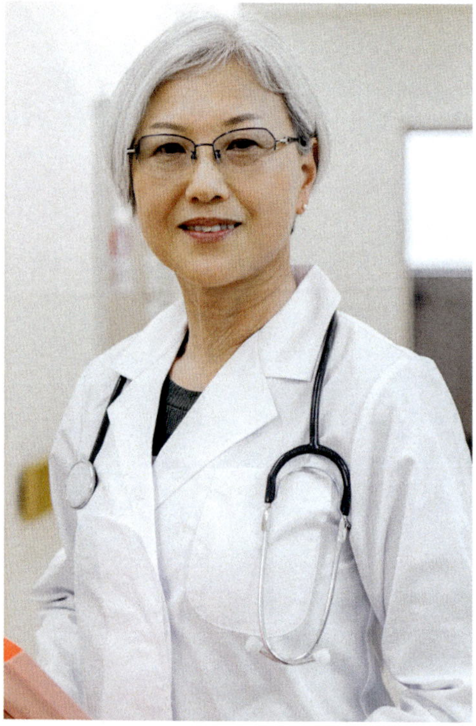
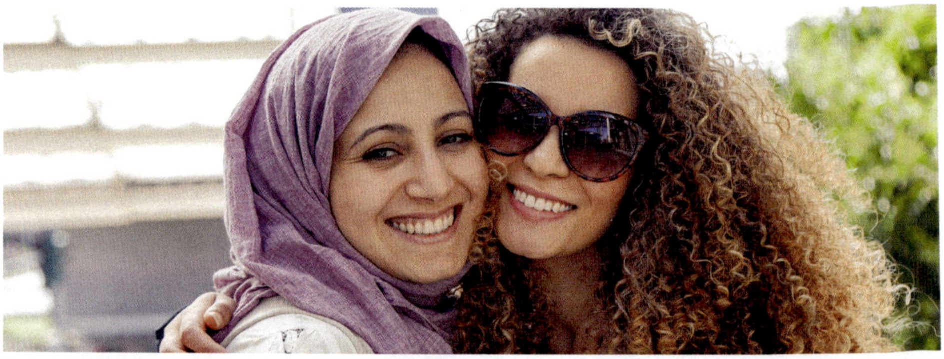
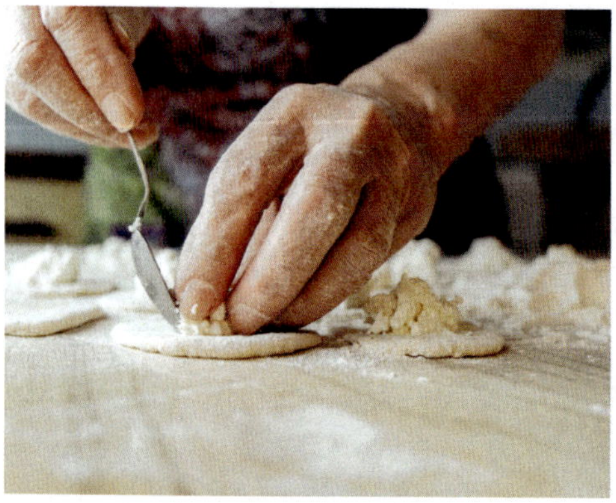
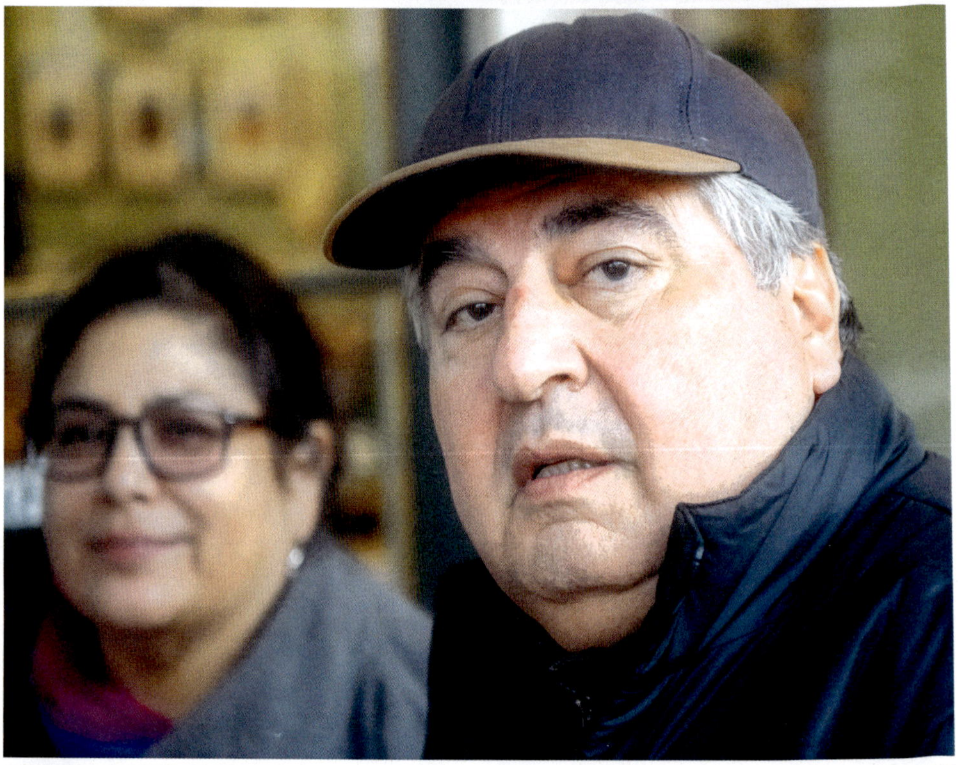
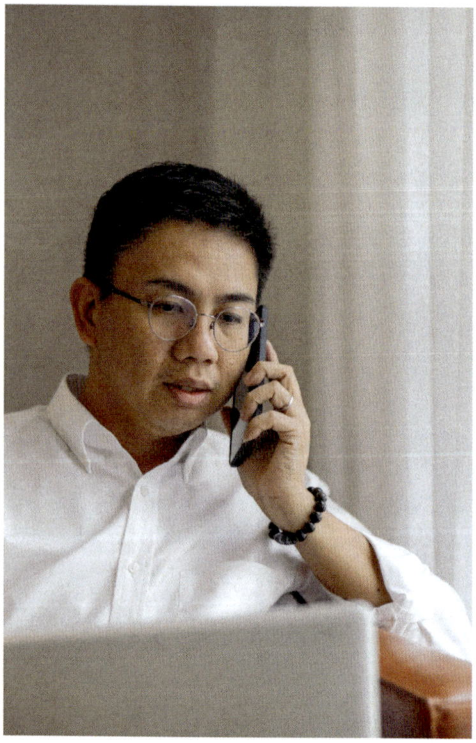
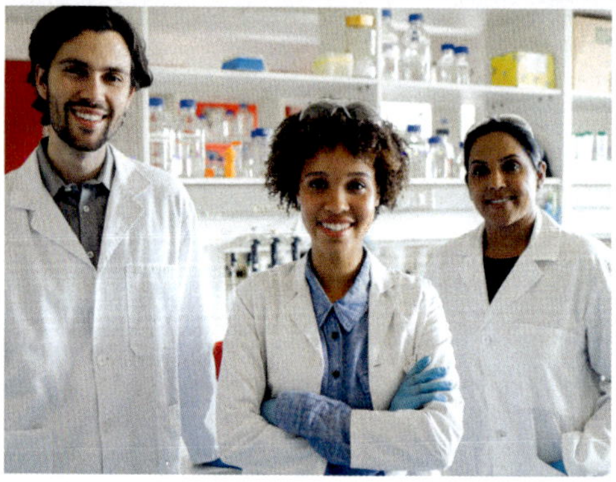
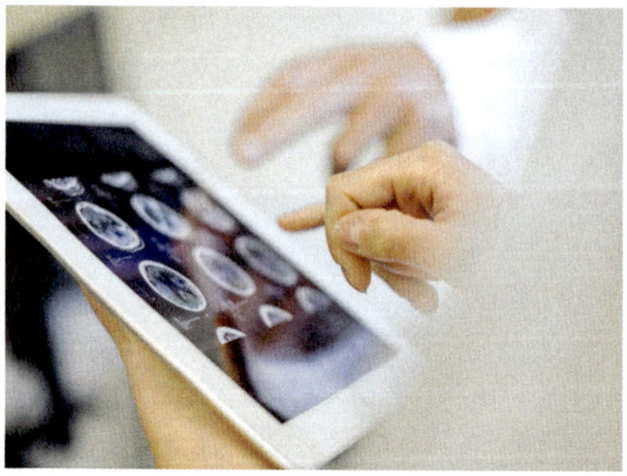
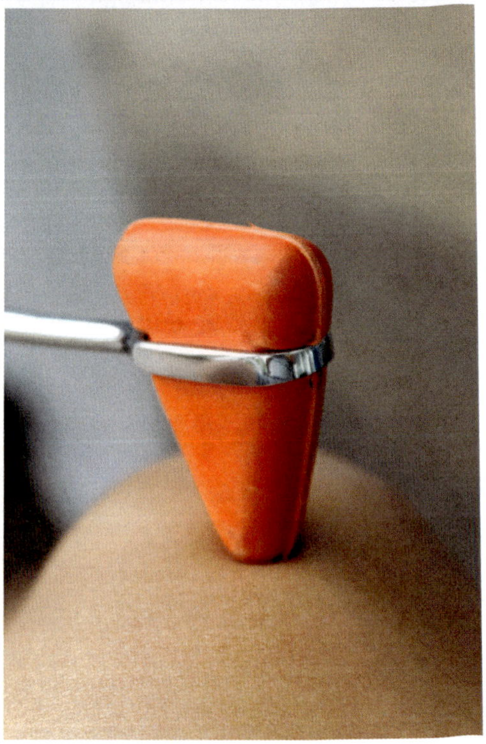

Contents

1
About CAR T-cell therapy

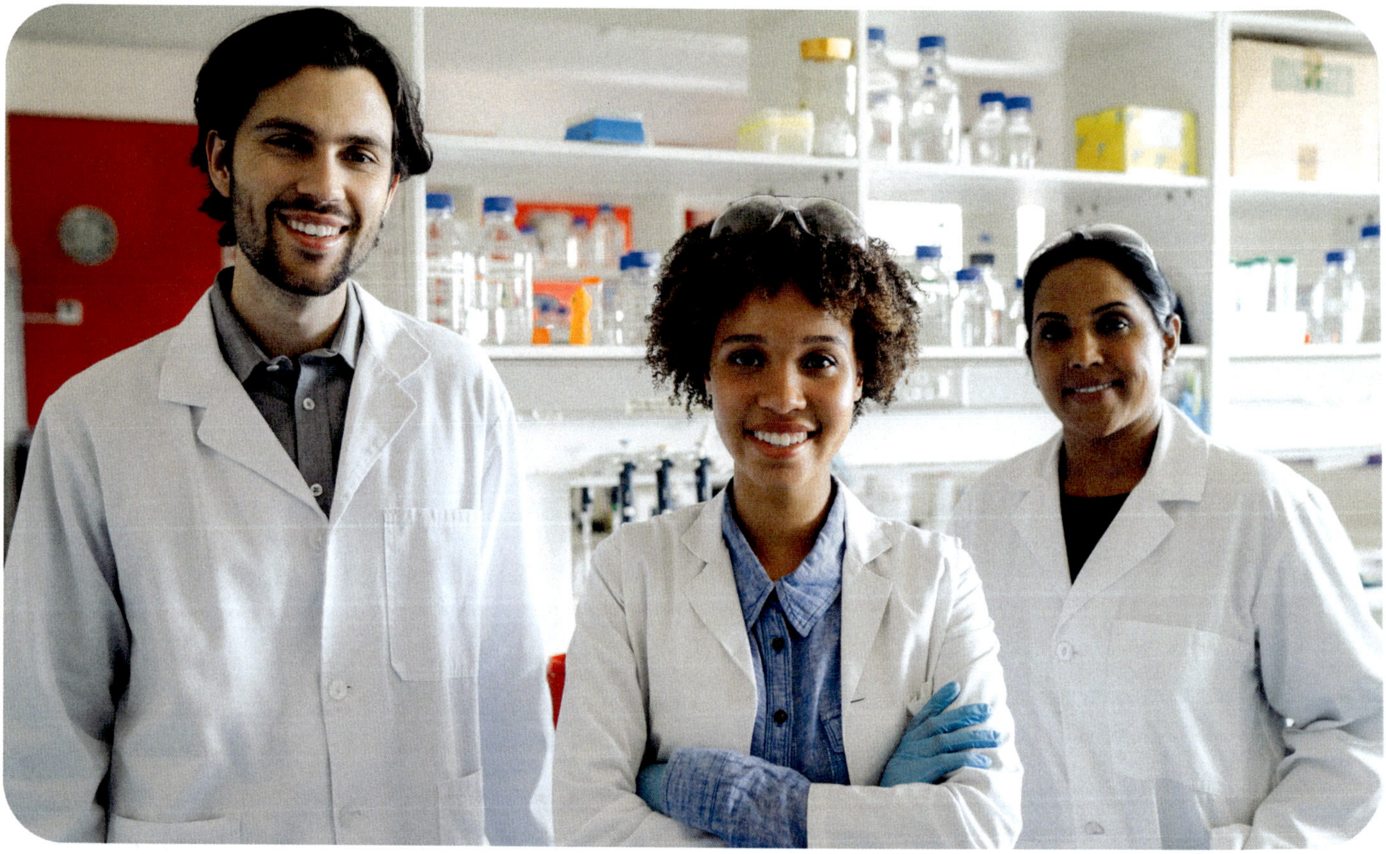

What is CAR T-cell therapy?

CAR T-cell therapy is a new type of immunotherapy. Immunotherapy is an approach to cancer treatment that harnesses the power of the immune system to kill cancer cells. There are now many different ways to use the immune system against cancer. In addition to CAR T-cell therapy, other types of immunotherapy include:

- Immune checkpoint inhibitors (ICIs)
- Antibodies
- Cancer vaccines
- Oncolytic virus therapy

Some immunotherapies play an indirect role in killing cancer cells, such as by helping normal immune cells better recognize cancer cells. Other types, including CAR T, work by re-engineering components of the immune system to attack cancer cells head-on.

In the CAR-T manufacturing process, immune cells are sent to a laboratory where they are "armed" with a special receptor. This receptor—called chimeric antigen receptor (CAR)—guides immune cells to find and kill cancer cells using a "search and destroy" approach.

The CAR T process

White blood cells called T cells, or T lymphocytes, are taken from your blood. In the CAR-T manufacturing facility, the CAR gene is introduced into the cells, making them "CAR T cells." This makes CAR T a gene therapy in addition to an immunotherapy. Another name for CAR T cells is immune effector cells (IECs). Next, the CAR T cells are grown in mass quantities. After you receive a short course of chemotherapy, they are put back into your bloodstream. These millions of CAR T cells find and bind to cancer cells, killing them.

Currently available CAR T therapies

At this time there are two CAR T-cell therapies approved by the U.S. Food & Drug Administration (FDA) for cancer treatment:

- Axicabtagene ciloleucel (Yescarta®)
- Tisagenlecleucel (Kymriah®)

Both bind to a protein called CD19, which is found on some leukemia cells and most B-cell lymphoma cells. They are both approved to treat several forms of B-cell non-Hodgkin lymphomas (NHLs). Kymriah® is also approved to treat B-cell acute lymphoblastic leukemia (ALL).

Yescarta® and Kymriah® are usually only used to treat cancer that does not respond to other treatment, or that has returned after treatment.

Serious side effects

CAR T-cell therapy is an aggressive cancer treatment. Severe and potentially life-threatening effects are possible, including:

- Cytokine release syndrome (CRS)
- Neurologic (nervous system-related) problems together known as immune effector cell-associated neurotoxicity syndrome (ICANS)

CRS is the focus of the next chapter; neurologic effects are discussed in Chapter 3.

The U.S. FDA requires that manufacturers of drugs with very serious risks develop a Risk

Evaluation and Mitigation Strategy (REMS). The purpose of a REMS is to ensure that the benefits of a drug outweigh its potential risks and that providers are fully educated in the management of CAR-T side effects. The FDA has determined that a REMS is necessary for both Yescarta® and Kymriah®.

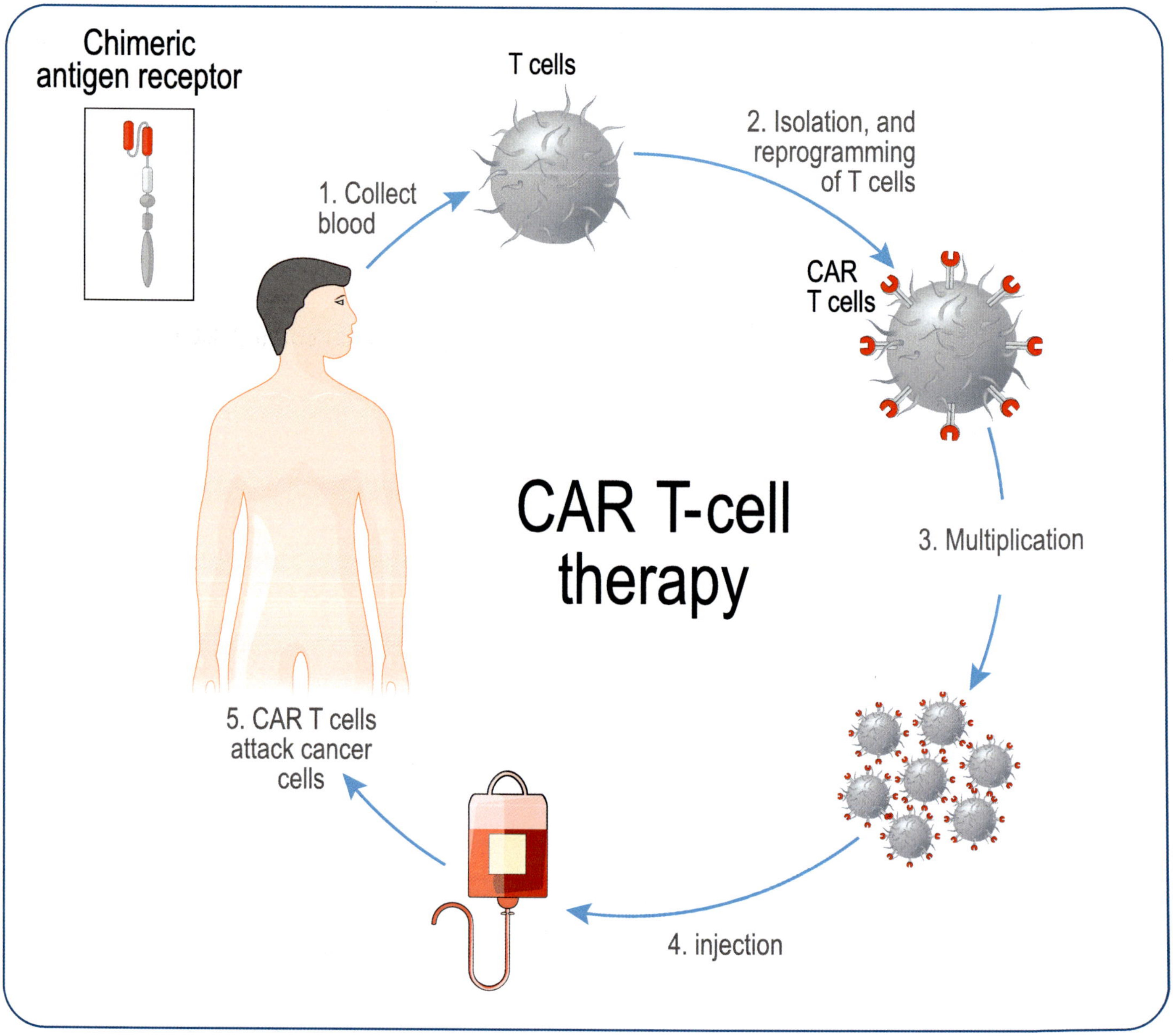

Before and during infusion

Central venous access

Yescarta® and Kymriah® are given intravenously. This means they are put directly into the bloodstream through a vein. A type of catheter called a central venous catheter is often used when long-term (weeks or months) vein access is needed.

A thin tube is inserted into your vein, usually below the collarbone or in the upper arm. The tube is guided into the superior vena cava vein, a large vein above the right side of the heart. When needed, this catheter will be accessed to draw blood, give fluids, or administer CAR T-cell therapy.

Tumor lysis syndrome

Cancer cells break apart when they die. The contents of the dead cancer cells enter the bloodstream and disrupt the chemical balance of the blood. This is called tumor lysis syndrome (TLS). This potentially dangerous side effect of cancer treatment can lead to organ damage and be life-threatening. TLS most often occurs after treatment of aggressive (fast-growing) cancers. Your physician may use medications to prevent or treat TLS if it occurs.

Preventing seizures

You may receive medication to prevent seizures before an infusion of CAR T-cell therapy. A medication called levetiracetam is commonly used for this purpose. It is an anti-convulsant. Anti-convulsants reduce abnormal overactivity in the brain. Levetiracetam is usually taken as a pill every 12 hours for up to 30 days. Other medications may be used in place of levetiracetam at the discretion of your treatment team.

After CAR T-cell therapy

Most people stay in the hospital for at least a week after CAR T-cell therapy. This allows for close monitoring and treatment of urgent side effects. Early signs of CRS or nervous system problems will be easier to spot while being monitored in the hospital.

If hospital (inpatient) care is not possible, close monitoring by a center with CAR T outpatient experience may be an option. If CRS or nervous system side effects occur, hospitalization is usually necessary.

Blood and laboratory testing

You will have ongoing blood testing while in the hospital to monitor for any deficiencies or problems. Blood tests you are likely to have include:

- Complete blood count (CBC)
- Comprehensive metabolic panel (CMP)
- Coagulation profile
- C-reactive protein (CRP)
- Ferritin

Long-term side effects

Low blood cell counts

For weeks to months after CAR T-cell therapy you may have lower-than-normal numbers of red blood cells, white blood cells, and platelets. Having low blood cell counts increases your risk of infection. One or both of the following may be used to try to minimize risk of infection:

- Blood and platelet transfusions
- Growth factors

Your doctor may recommend a blood transfusion to raise your levels of red blood cells and/or platelets. In a transfusion, cells donated by healthy volunteers are put into your bloodstream through a vein. Transfusions are not typically used to treat low white blood cell counts.

Growth factors are medications that stimulate the bone marrow to produce more blood cells. They are given by injection or intravenously. Erythropoiesis-stimulating agents (ESAs) can help your body produce more red blood cells. Colony-stimulating growth factors such as filgrastim (Neupogen®) can also help your body produce more white blood cells.

Low numbers of B cells

CAR T-cell therapy is most often used to treat B-cell non-Hodgkin lymphomas (NHLs). In the process of killing the bad B cells with cancer, normal B cells are destroyed. Having low numbers of B cells is called B-cell aplasia. This is a normal, long-term side effect of CAR T therapy. Having too few B cells is a good sign. It means that the CAR T cells continue to fight the cancer.

However, it also means that you have fewer antibodies (also called immunoglobulins) to protect you from infection. This creates a condition called hypogammaglobulinemia. You may have treatment to boost your antibody levels. This is called immunoglobulin replacement therapy. In immunoglobulin replacement therapy, you are given one or more infusions of a mixture of antibodies. These donated antibodies can help strengthen your immune system and fight infection.

Review

- CAR T-cell therapy is a newer form of immunotherapy in which immune cells are re-engineered in a laboratory and put back into the body.
- The re-engineered immune cells–now armed with a special receptor–find and kill cancer cells using a "search and destroy" approach.
- You may receive medication to prevent seizures before receiving CAR T-cell therapy.
- Most people stay at the hospital for at least a week after receiving CAR T. This allows for close monitoring and treatment of urgent side effects.
- The most common side effect of CAR T-cell therapy is cytokine release syndrome (CRS).
- The neurologic (nervous system-related) problems that can occur after CAR T-cell therapy are together known as immune effector cell-associated neurotoxicity syndrome (ICANS).
- Low blood cell counts are common after CAR T-cell therapy. You may receive blood transfusions and/or growth factors to help prevent infection.
- Having low numbers of B cells is called B-cell aplasia. It is a normal, long-term side effect of CAR T therapy.
- Immunoglobulin replacement therapy may be used to strengthen your immune system and fight infection after CAR T-cell therapy.

2

Cytokine release syndrome (CRS)

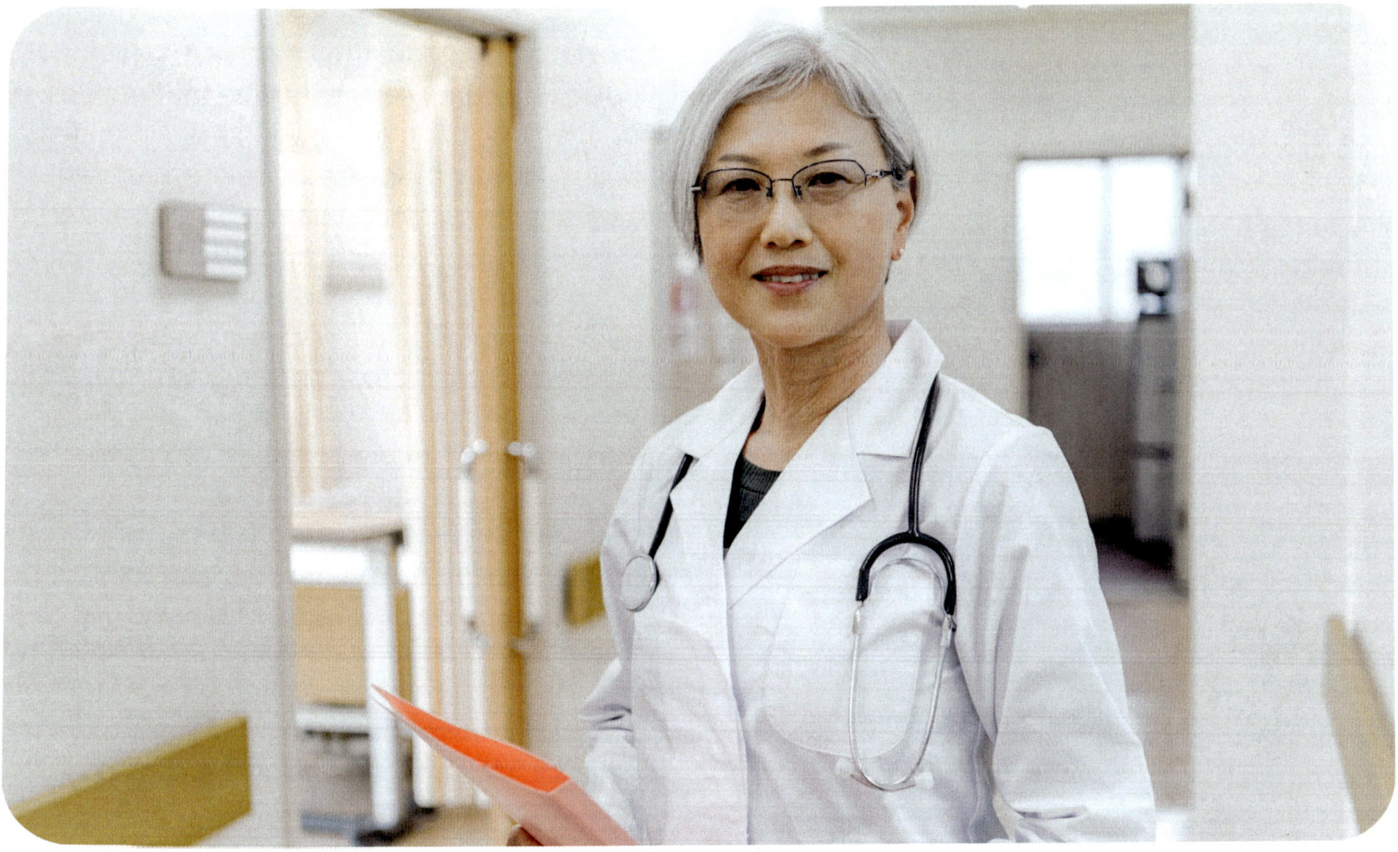

The majority of patients experience cytokine release syndrome (CRS) after CAR T-cell therapy. It is the most common, serious side effect of CAR T. Although CRS is often mild, it can be severe.

What is CRS?

Cytokines are proteins that carry out different immune-related jobs in the body. Some types contribute to inflammation (pro-inflammatory cytokines) while others help to reduce it (anti-inflammatory cytokines).

In the days following an infusion of CAR T-cell therapy, immune cells affected by the treatment may release pro-inflammatory cytokines into the blood. The cytokines stimulate an inflammatory response, called cytokine release syndrome (CRS). Symptoms of CRS include fever, chills, low blood pressure, rapid heartbeat, trouble breathing, and low oxygen, among others. See Guide 1.

While most patients experience CRS, you do not need to experience it for CAR T cells to work. Your cancer type and the specific CAR T medicine you are treated with both play a role in how likely you are to experience CRS.

CRS generally starts 2 to 3 days after receiving an infusion of CAR T-cell therapy and lasts about a week (7 to 8 days). CRS can result in damage to major organs, including the heart, liver, kidneys, and lungs.

Serious CRS events

While most patients experience only mild CRS, serious and life-threatening complications are possible.

Low blood pressure

Blood pressure is the strength of your blood pushing against the sides of your blood vessels. CRS can cause your blood pressure to drop. Low blood pressure is dangerous because it reduces blood flow to the heart, brain, and other vital organs. In severe cases, low blood pressure can be life-threatening.

Vasopressors are a group of medicines that raise blood pressure by contracting (tightening) blood vessels. They are used in emergency situations to treat severely low blood pressure. Common vasopressors include norepinephrine, epinephrine, vasopressin, and dopamine.

Low tissue oxygen levels (hypoxia)

Hypoxia is a dangerous condition that happens when there isn't enough oxygen reaching the cells and tissues of the body. Your brain, liver, and other organs can be damaged in a matter of minutes if they don't receive enough oxygen.

Oxygen therapy is used to ensure that your tissues and organs are getting enough oxygen. Depending on how low your tissue oxygen level is, you may receive oxygen through noninvasive nose tubes (nasal cannula) or a mask that covers your nose and mouth. In severe cases, intubation may be necessary. Intubation refers to putting a tube, called an endotracheal tube, through the mouth and into the airway. The endotracheal tube is connected to a respirator that moves air in and out of your lungs. This is called mechanical ventilation.

Other serious events

Heart (cardiac) effects

CRS can cause heart rhythm problems (cardiac arrhythmias). The heart may beat more quickly, more slowly, or at irregular intervals. Atrial fibrillation ("a-fib") refers to a rapid and irregular heartbeat. In ventricular tachycardia or "V-tack" the heart beats quickly but at even intervals (regularly). Abnormal heart rhythms can be dangerous and may require additional medications and treatment to manage.

CRS can also cause decreased heart performance, but this is often temporary. Sudden cardiac arrest is also possible, but is not common.

Poor kidney function

CRS may increase the risk of acute kidney injury (AKI) after CAR T-cell therapy. However, this is not common and the effects are usually reversible (not permanent) for most people.

Capillary leak syndrome

Capillary leak syndrome is a condition in which fluid and proteins leak out of the bloodstream through tiny blood vessels (capillaries). It can lead to dangerously low blood pressure, multiple organ failure, and shock.

Macrophage activation syndrome

A macrophage is a type of white blood cell that kills viruses and bacteria, gets rid of dead cells, and stimulates the action of other immune cells. Macrophage activation syndrome (MAS) is a hyper-inflammatory condition in which too many macrophages and T cells are made by the body. In MAS, the body becomes flooded with inflammatory cytokines and may lead to serious organ damage.

Guide 1 Signs and symptoms of CRS
Low blood pressure (hypotension)
Low tissue oxygen level (hypoxia)
Fever
Chills
Rapid heartbeat
Nausea
Rash
Headache
Trouble breathing

Treatments for CRS

Tocilizumab (Actemra®)

Interleukin-6, or IL-6, is a cytokine that is released during CRS, leading to very high levels of it in the blood. Tocilizumab is a prescription medicine that inhibits, or blocks, IL-6. Tocilizumab is essential to the treatment of moderate to severe CRS. It is also used to treat milder CRS in patients who have both neurologic (nervous system-related) toxicity and CRS.

Tocilizumab is given intravenously for the treatment of CRS. If there is no improvement after your first dose, up to three more doses may be given. Doses should be given at least 8 hours apart. No more than three doses of tocilizumab can be given in 24 hours.

Corticosteroids

Corticosteroids are medicines commonly used to relieve inflammation. They are used in combination with tocilizumab for the treatment of moderate to severe CRS. Dexamethasone and methylprednisolone are commonly used corticosteroids.

Review

- Cytokines are proteins that carry out different immune-related jobs in the body. Some contribute to inflammation and others help reduce it.
- CRS is the release of inflammation-causing cytokines into the blood after an infusion of CAR T-cell therapy.
- Signs and symptoms of CRS include fever, chills, rapid heartbeat, low blood pressure, nausea, rash, headache, and trouble breathing.
- Tocilizumab (Actemra®) is used to treat moderate to severe CRS. Corticosteroids are used in combination with tocilizumab.
- The majority of patients experience CRS. It is overall the most common serious side effect of CAR T-cell therapy. Although CRS is often mild, it can be severe.

3 Neurologic toxicities

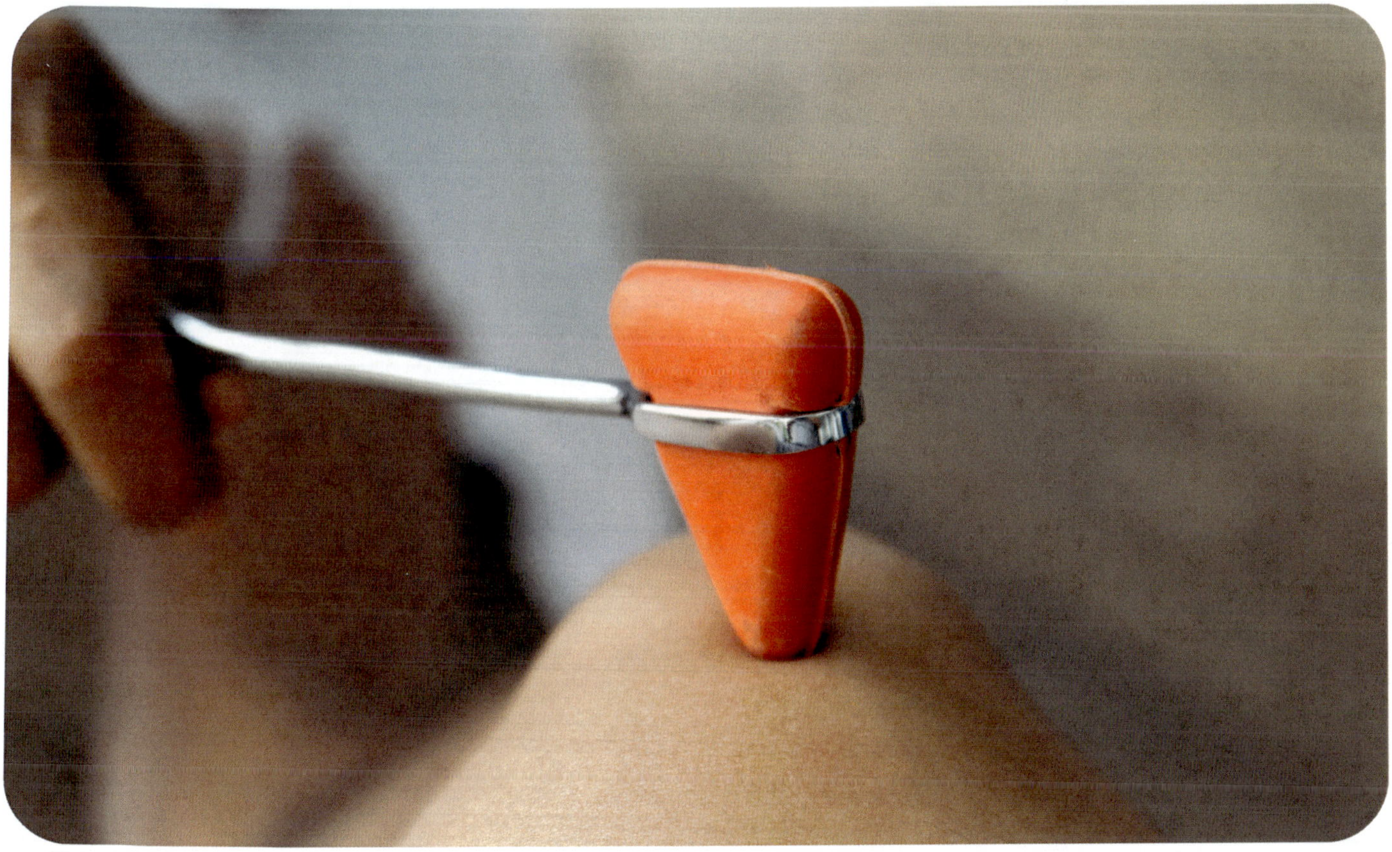

The neurologic (nervous system-related) side effects of CAR T-cell therapy range from mild to life-threatening. These effects are usually reversible if treated promptly.

What are neurologic toxicities?

The brain and nervous system problems that can occur after CAR T-cell therapy are called neurotoxicities. Common, mild symptoms include headache, dizziness, trouble sleeping, shaking (tremor), confusion, memory issues, and anxiety. In more severe cases, seizures, brain swelling, and coma can occur and may be life-threatening. See Guide 2.

Most of the possible nervous system symptoms are together known as immune effector cell-associated neurotoxicity syndrome (ICANS). Your doctors use an ICANS grading system to determine how severe your symptoms are.

Neurologic side effects typically start 4 to 10 days after treatment and last about 2 weeks, although they can last as long as 4 to 8 weeks.

Delirium

Delirium is a sudden change in brain function that causes confusion, disorientation, and changes in behavior or emotions. It can also cause agitation, hallucinations, and extreme excitement. Delirium comes on quickly, typically in a matter of hours to days.

Nerve dysfunction

Your autonomic nervous system is constantly working behind the scenes to regulate your basic body functions, including your heart rate, digestion, breathing rate, and body temperature.

ICANS can lead to autonomic nervous system dysfunction, causing symptoms such as dizziness upon standing up (orthostatic hypotension), sweating too much or too little, and digestive and urinary problems.

Language impairment (aphasia)

Aphasia is the loss of ability to understand or express speech, caused by brain damage. It is a language disorder. Aphasia does not affect your intelligence. People with aphasia are still able to formulate thoughts in the same way, but are unable to communicate them as they did before. This can be very frustrating.

Guide 2 Brain and nervous system effects
Headache
Shaking (tremor)
Dizziness
Insomnia
Anxiety
Language impairment (aphasia)
Delirium
Nerve dysfunction (autonomic neuropathy)
Seizures
Brain damage (encephalopathy)

Serious complications

While not common, serious and potentially life-threatening nervous system problems can occur after CAR T-cell therapy.

Seizures

Abnormal electrical signals in the brain can cause sudden and uncontrolled body movements, shaking in particular. These are called seizures. Other symptoms of seizures include behavior changes, loss of awareness, and loss of muscle control.

Convulsive status epilepticus is the medical term for having one long (5 minutes or more) seizure, or several shorter seizures in a row. Convulsive status epilepticus is a medical emergency that can occur in severe ICANS.

You will receive care according to the protocols at the hospital where you are being treated. Hospital treatment of convulsive status epilepticus typically includes use of several different types of drugs, given in a specific order.

Brain swelling

Swelling due to trapped fluid—also called edema—is the body's response to many types of injury and illness. Swelling of the brain (cerebral edema) is a life-threatening inflammatory reaction to CAR T-cell therapy. When the brain swells, it increases the pressure inside the skull (intracranial pressure).

Osmotic therapy is the use of medicines to draw cerebrospinal fluid out of the skull and fluid out of the injured brain, reducing pressure. Another name for osmotic therapy is hyperosmolar therapy. The most commonly used osmotic drugs are hypertonic saline and mannitol.

In severe cases of brain swelling, surgery may be necessary. Surgery could involve removing a part of the skull and repairing any damage. Another possible procedure is called

Monitoring for seizures

You may have electroencephalography (EEG) to monitor for seizures during ICANS. An EEG is a recording of electrical activity in the brain.

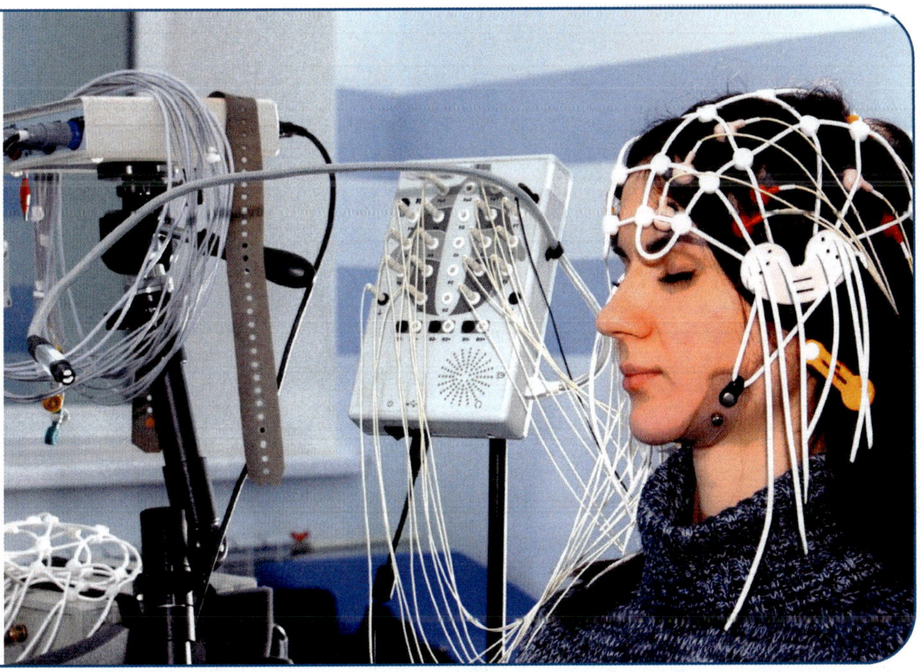

a ventriculostomy. It involves inserting a plastic tube into the skull to drain excess fluid in order to lower the pressure.

How severe is it?

Doctors use a point system to rate the seriousness of sudden nervous system events after CAR T-cell therapy.

The Immune Effector Cell-Associated Encephalopathy (ICE) Assessment Tool is a brain damage screening test. It provides a snapshot of your overall mental state and your ability to carry out simple tasks, such as writing and counting. A score of 0 (critical emergency) to 10 (mild) is possible.

In addition to your ICE score, the following information is used to determine the overall severity of ICANS:

- How alert/responsive you are
- Whether you are experiencing seizures
- Whether you have any significant muscle weakness
- Whether there is brain swelling

This information is used to assign ICANS a grade from 1 to 4, with 4 being the most severe (life-threatening). The grades help guide treatment decisions.

This grading system was developed by the American Society of Blood and Marrow Transplantation, now the American Society for Transplantation and Cellular Therapy (ASTCT).

Lumbar puncture

A lumbar puncture may be needed if ICANS becomes severe. The purpose is to remove and test cerebrospinal fluid (CSF).

Reproduced with permission by Blausen.com staff (2014). "Medical gallery of Blausen Medical 2014". WikiJournal of Medicine 1 (2). DOI:10.15347/wjm/2014.010. ISSN 2002-4436.Wikimedia Commons.

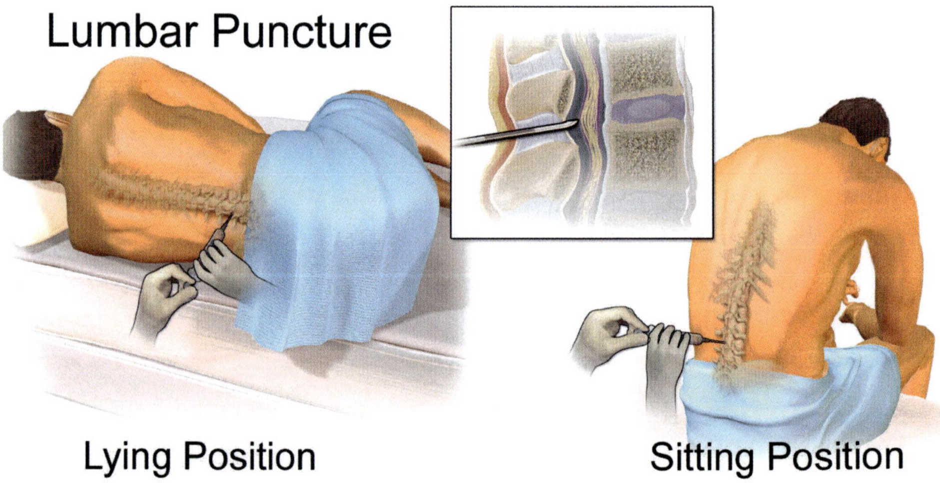

Treatments for neurotoxicity

Supportive care may be all that is needed for mild ICANS. Intravenous corticosteroids are used to treat moderate and severe ICANS. Corticosteroids are medicines commonly used to relieve inflammation. Dexamethasone and methylprednisolone are commonly used corticosteroids.

If you also have CRS

If you also have cytokine release syndrome, you will receive anti-IL-6 therapy with tocilizumab (Actemra®) as an additional treatment. No more than three doses should be given in 24 hours.

Assessment and supportive care

Other testing and care you may have while in the hospital are described next.

Neurologic assessment

You will have frequent neurologic assessments while in the hospital. These exams will check your mental status, motor function, and look for other signs of brain and nervous system problems.

Supportive care

You may receive fluids intravenously (an "IV drip") to keep you hydrated. You care team will also take steps to prevent food or liquid from going into your airway instead of your esophagus. This is called aspiration. Aspiration can lead to infection, particularly pneumonia and lung inflammation (pneumonitis).

Monitoring for seizures

You may have monitoring for seizures. An electroencephalogram (EEG) is used to detect seizure activity. An EEG is a recording of electrical activity in the brain. It tracks and records brain wave patterns transmitted by small metal sensors placed on your scalp.

Brain imaging

You may have magnetic resonance imaging (MRI) of your brain. If an MRI is not possible, you may have computed tomography (CT) instead.

Preventing infection

Corticosteroids are used for moderate and severe ICANS. Steroid therapy can weaken your immune system, making it easier for you to get an infection. Your doctor may prescribe medication to prevent fungal infections, such as fluconazole (Diflucan®).

Lumbar puncture

If you have severe ICANS, you may have a lumbar puncture to confirm the diagnosis. A lumbar puncture is sometimes also ordered for moderate ICANS.

Review

- The nervous system side effects of CAR T-cell therapy are called neurotoxicities. They include immune effector cell-associated neurotoxicity syndrome (ICANS) and some other symptoms.
- Common symptoms include headache, dizziness, trouble sleeping, shaking (tremor), and anxiety.
- Delirium, language impairment (aphasia), and nerve dysfunction are also possible.
- Serious and life-threatening nervous system events include seizures, brain swelling, and coma. These effects are usually reversible.
- Supportive care may be all that is needed for mild ICANS.
- Intravenous corticosteroid therapy is used to treat moderate to severe ICANS.
- Tocilizumab (Actemra®) is given as an additional single-dose therapy for people with both ICANS and CRS.

4 Resources

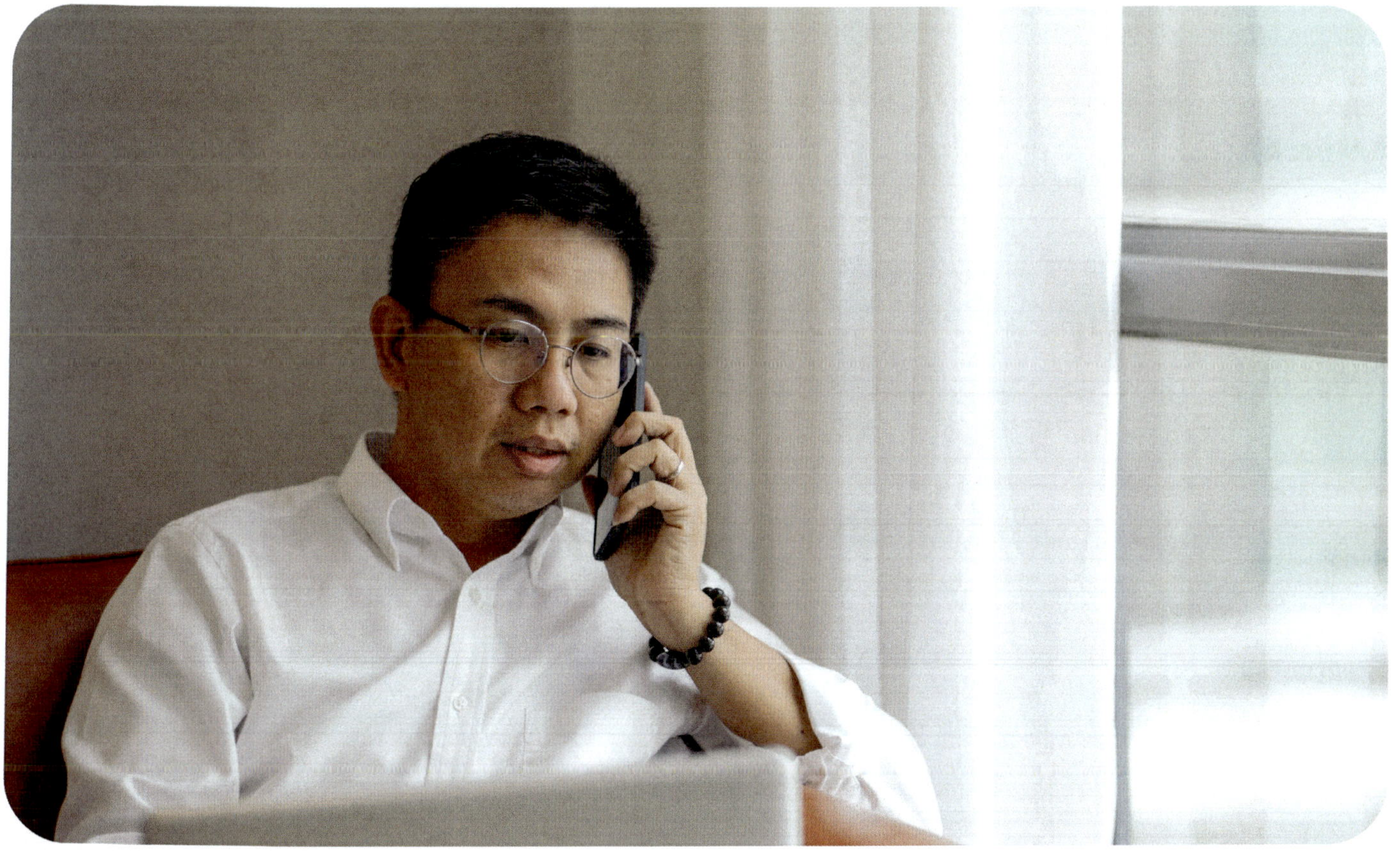

CAR T-cell therapy is a recent and promising innovation in cancer treatment. This chapter includes resources for learning more about this type of immunotherapy and its effects.

Questions to ask your doctor

It is normal to have lots of questions about immunotherapy with CAR T-cell therapy. Possible questions to ask your doctor are listed on the following pages. Feel free to use these questions or come up with your own.

Following the questions is a listing of websites that provide information for patients about CAR T-cell therapy and its effects.

Your health care provider may provide you with a wallet card that states the type of immunotherapy you are receiving, potential side effects, and contact numbers for your cancer care team. Carry it with you at all times.

Finding a clinical trial

- Search the National Institutes of Health (NIH) database for clinical trials. It includes publicly and privately funded clinical trials, whom to contact, and how to enroll. Look for an open clinical trial for your specific type of cancer. Go to **ClinicalTrials.gov**.
- The National Cancer Institute's Cancer Information Service (CIS) provides up-to-date information on clinical trials. You can call, e-mail, or chat live. Call 1.800.4.CANCER (800.422.6237) or go to **cancer.gov**.

Questions to ask your doctor about CAR T-cell therapy

1. Am I a candidate for immunotherapy with CAR T-cell therapy?
2. How is CAR T-cell therapy different from chemotherapy?
3. Where is CAR T-cell therapy available? Do I have to join a clinical trial?
4. Will my insurance cover CAR T-cell therapy?
5. What is the treatment process for patients? How long is the process?
6. Do I need chemotherapy before CAR T-cell therapy? Why?
7. How long do I need to stay in the hospital after CAR T-cell therapy? Can I just be monitored from home instead?
8. What are the side effects of CAR T-cell therapy? When do they start? How long do they usually last? How are they treated?
9. What are the chances of remission or cure?
10. How can I learn more about CAR T-cell therapy?

Websites

American Cancer Society
https://www.cancer.org/treatment/treatments-and-side-effects/treatment-types/immunotherapy/car-t-cell1.html

Be the Match®
BeTheMatch.org/one-on-one

Good Days
mygooddays.org

Lymphoma Research Foundation
https://lymphoma.org/aboutlymphoma/treatments/cartcell/

Oncology Nursing Society
Immunotherapy Wallet Cards
https://www.ons.org/sites/default/files/2019-01/IO%20Card%201-sided_Vertical.pdf

Society for Immunotherapy of Cancer
Understanding Cancer Immunotherapy, 5th *Edition*
https://www.sitcancer.org/HigherLogic/System/DownloadDocumentFile.ashx?DocumentFileKey=567abb47-c7f1-2fa3-b008-053953020940&forceDialog=0

Stupid Cancer
stupidcancer.org

The Leukemia & Lymphoma Society
lls.org/informationspecialists

U.S. National Library of Medicine
Clinical Trials Database
clinicaltrials.gov

Words to know

Actemra®
A prescription medicine used to treat severe or life-threatening cytokine release syndrome caused by CAR T-cell therapy. Also called tocilizumab.

aphasia
A language disorder caused by brain damage. A possible neurologic side effect of CAR T-cell therapy.

B-cell aplasia
Having low numbers of B cells. A normal, long-term side effect of CAR T-cell therapy.

capillary leak syndrome
The escape of fluid and proteins from blood vessels into surrounding tissues, resulting in dangerously low blood pressure.

cerebral edema
Brain swelling that causes an increase in intracranial pressure. A possible side effect of CAR T-cell therapy.

chimeric antigen receptor (CAR) T-cell therapy
A type of immunotherapy in which T cells (a type of immune system cell) are changed in the laboratory so they will attack cancer cells.

convulsive status epilepticus
A seizure lasting longer than 5 minutes, or having multiple seizures within a 5-minute period without fully recovering between them.

corticosteroids
Inflammation-reducing medicines. They lessen swelling, redness, itching, and allergic reactions. Used to treat side effects of CAR T-cell therapy.

cytokine release syndrome (CRS)
A potentially serious side effect of CAR T-cell therapy. Caused by the release of inflammatory proteins into the blood from immune cells affected by the immunotherapy.

delirium
A mental state causing confusion, disorientation, and memory problems. May also cause agitation, hallucinations, and extreme excitement. A possible side effect of CAR T-cell therapy.

hypogammaglobulinemia
An immune system problem in which not enough antibodies are made, resulting in increased infection risk.

hypotension
Low blood pressure. A possible complication of cytokine release syndrome.

hypoxia
Decreased oxygen supply to body tissue. A possible complication of cytokine release syndrome.

immune effector cell-associated neurotoxicity syndrome (ICANS)
A group of neurologic (nervous system-related) side effects of CAR T-cell therapy.

immunoglobulin replacement therapy
Treatment to increase antibody (immune globulin) levels. A solution made from antibodies taken from the blood of healthy donors is given through a vein. Also called intravenous immune globulin (IVIG).

Kymriah®
A CAR T-cell therapy used to treat B-cell cancers that have not responded to other treatment or that have returned after treatment. Also called tisagenlecleucel.

macrophage activation syndrome (MAS)
A condition in which too many of a type of white blood cell (macrophage) and T cells are made by the body. The body becomes flooded with inflammatory cytokines and may lead to serious organ damage.

osmotic therapy
The use of medicines to draw cerebrospinal fluid out of the skull and fluid out of the brain, reducing pressure. Also called hyperosmolar therapy.

Risk Evaluation and Mitigation Strategy (REMS)
A strategy to ensure that the benefits of using a drug outweigh its very serious potential risks. Required by the U.S. Food & Drug Administration (FDA) for currently available CAR T-cell therapies.

seizure
Sudden, uncontrolled body movements and changes in behavior caused by abnormal electrical activity in the brain.

tumor lysis syndrome (TLS)
A condition that can occur after treatment of a fast-growing cancer, especially certain blood cancers. As tumor cells die, they break apart and release their contents into the blood. This causes a change in certain chemicals in the blood, which may cause organ damage.

vasopressor
Medicine that raises blood pressure by contracting (tightening) blood vessels. Used in emergency situations to treat severely low blood pressure.

Yescarta®
A CAR T-cell therapy used to treat B-cell cancers that have not responded to other treatment or that have returned after treatment. Also called axicabtagene ciloleucel.

NCCN Contributors

This patient guide is based on the NCCN Clinical Practice Guidelines in Oncology (NCCN Guidelines®) for Management of Immunotherapy-Related Toxicities. It was adapted, reviewed, and published with help from the following people:

Dorothy A. Shead, MS
Director, Patient Information Operations

Laura J. Hanisch, PsyD
Medical Writer/Patient Information Specialist

Erin Vidic, MA
Medical Writer

Rachael Clarke
Senior Medical Copyeditor

Tanya Fischer, MEd, MSLIS
Medical Writer

Kim Williams
Creative Services Manager

Susan Kidney
Design Specialist

The NCCN Clinical Practice Guidelines in Oncology (NCCN Guidelines®) for Management of Immunotherapy-Related Toxicities (Version 1.2020, December 16, 2019) were developed by the following NCCN Panel Members:

John A. Thompson, MD/Chair
Fred Hutchinson Cancer Research Center/ Seattle Cancer Care Alliance

Bryan J. Schneider, MD/Vice-Chair
University of Michigan Rogel Cancer Center

Julie Brahmer, MD/Vice-Chair
The Sidney Kimmel Comprehensive Cancer Center at Johns Hopkins

Stephanie Andrews, MS, ANP-BC
Moffitt Cancer Center

Philippe Armand, MD, PhD*
Dana-Farber/Brigham and Women's Cancer Center

Shailender Bhatia, MD
Fred Hutchinson Cancer Research Center/ Seattle Cancer Care Alliance

Lihua E. Budde, MD, PhD*
City of Hope National Medical Center

Luciano Costa, MD, PhD
O'Neal Comprehensive Cancer Center at UAB

Marianne Davies, DNP, RN, AOCNP
Yale Cancer Center/Smilow Cancer Hospital

David Dunnington, MA
Patient Advocate

Marc S. Ernstoff, MD
Roswell Park Comprehensive Cancer Center

Matthew Frigault, MD*
Massachusetts General Hospital Cancer Center

Benjamin H. Kaffenberger
The Ohio State University Comprehensive Cancer Center - James Cancer Hospital and Solove Research Institute

Matthew Lunning, DO
Fred & Pamela Buffett Cancer Center

Suzanne McGettigan, MSN, CRNP
Abramson Cancer Center at the University of Pennsylvania

Jordan McPherson, PharmD, MS, BCOP
Huntsman Cancer Institute at the University of Utah

Nisha A. Mohindra, MD
Robert H. Lurie Comprehensive Cancer Center of Northwestern University

Jarushka Naidoo, MD
The Sidney Kimmel Comprehensive Cancer Center at Johns Hopkins

Anthony J. Olszanski, MD, RPh
Fox Chase Cancer Center

Olalekan Oluwole, MD
Vanderbilt-Ingram Cancer Center

Sandip P. Patel, MD
UC San Diego Moores Cancer Center

Nathan Pennell, MD, PhD
Case Comprehensive Cancer Center/ University Hospitals Seidman Cancer Center and Cleveland Clinic Taussig Cancer Institute

Sunil Reddy, MD
Stanford Cancer Institute

Mabel Ryder, MD
Mayo Clinic Cancer Center

Bianca Santomasso, MD, PhD
Memorial Sloan Kettering Cancer Center

Scott Shofer, MD, PhD
Duke Cancer Institute

Jeffrey A. Sosman, MD
Robert H. Lurie Comprehensive Cancer Center of Northwestern University

Yinghong Wang, MD, PhD
The University of Texas MD Anderson Cancer Center

Ryan M. Weight, DO, MS
University of Colorado Cancer Center

NCCN Staff

Alyse Johnson-Chilla, MSS
Guidelines Coordinator

* Reviewed this patient guide.
For disclosures, visit NCCN.org/about/disclosure.aspx.

NCCN Cancer Centers

Abramson Cancer Center
at the University of Pennsylvania
Philadelphia, Pennsylvania
800.789.7366 • pennmedicine.org/cancer

Fred & Pamela Buffett Cancer Center
Omaha, Nebraska
800.999.5465 • nebraskamed.com/cancer

Case Comprehensive Cancer Center/
University Hospitals Seidman Cancer
Center and Cleveland Clinic Taussig
Cancer Institute
Cleveland, Ohio
800.641.2422 • UH Seidman Cancer Center
uhhospitals.org/services/cancer-services
866.223.8100 • CC Taussig Cancer Institute
my.clevelandclinic.org/departments/cancer
216.844.8797 • Case CCC
case.edu/cancer

City of Hope National Medical Center
Los Angeles, California
800.826.4673 • cityofhope.org

Dana-Farber/Brigham and
Women's Cancer Center
Massachusetts General Hospital
Cancer Center
Boston, Massachusetts
877.332.4294
dfbwcc.org
massgeneral.org/cancer

Duke Cancer Institute
Durham, North Carolina
888.275.3853 • dukecancerinstitute.org

Fox Chase Cancer Center
Philadelphia, Pennsylvania
888.369.2427 • foxchase.org

Huntsman Cancer Institute
at the University of Utah
Salt Lake City, Utah
877.585.0303
huntsmancancer.org

Fred Hutchinson Cancer
Research Center/Seattle
Cancer Care Alliance
Seattle, Washington
206.288.7222 • seattlecca.org
206.667.5000 • fredhutch.org

The Sidney Kimmel Comprehensive
Cancer Center at Johns Hopkins
Baltimore, Maryland
410.955.8964
https://www.hopkinsmedicine.org/kimmel_cancer_center/

Robert H. Lurie Comprehensive
Cancer Center of Northwestern
University
Chicago, Illinois
866.587.4322 • cancer.northwestern.edu

Mayo Clinic Cancer Center
Phoenix/Scottsdale, Arizona
Jacksonville, Florida
Rochester, Minnesota
800.446.2279 • Arizona
904.953.0853 • Florida
507.538.3270 • Minnesota
mayoclinic.org/departments-centers/mayo-clinic-cancer-center

Memorial Sloan Kettering
Cancer Center
New York, New York
800.525.2225 • mskcc.org

Moffitt Cancer Center
Tampa, Florida
800.456.3434 • moffitt.org

The Ohio State University
Comprehensive Cancer Center -
James Cancer Hospital and
Solove Research Institute
Columbus, Ohio
800.293.5066 • cancer.osu.edu

O'Neal Comprehensive
Cancer Center at UAB
Birmingham, Alabama
800.822.0933 • uab.edu/onealcancercenter

Roswell Park Comprehensive
Cancer Center
Buffalo, New York
877.275.7724 • roswellpark.org

Siteman Cancer Center at Barnes-
Jewish Hospital and Washington
University School of Medicine
St. Louis, Missouri
800.600.3606 • siteman.wustl.edu

St. Jude Children's Research Hospital
The University of Tennessee
Health Science Center
Memphis, Tennessee
888.226.4343 • stjude.org
901.683.0055 • westclinic.com

Stanford Cancer Institute
Stanford, California
877.668.7535 • cancer.stanford.edu

UC San Diego Moores Cancer Center
La Jolla, California
858.657.7000 • cancer.ucsd.edu

UCLA Jonsson
Comprehensive Cancer Center
Los Angeles, California
310.825.5268 • cancer.ucla.edu

UCSF Helen Diller Family
Comprehensive Cancer Center
San Francisco, California
800.689.8273 • cancer.ucsf.edu

University of Colorado Cancer Center
Aurora, Colorado
720.848.0300 • coloradocancercenter.org

University of Michigan
Rogel Cancer Center
Ann Arbor, Michigan
800.865.1125 • rogelcancercenter.org

The University of Texas
MD Anderson Cancer Center
Houston, Texas
800.392.1611 • mdanderson.org

University of Wisconsin
Carbone Cancer Center
Madison, Wisconsin
608.265.1700 • uwhealth.org/cancer

UT Southwestern Simmons
Comprehensive Cancer Center
Dallas, Texas
214.648.3111 • utswmed.org/cancer

Vanderbilt-Ingram Cancer Center
Nashville, Tennessee
800.811.8480 • vicc.org

Yale Cancer Center/
Smilow Cancer Hospital
New Haven, Connecticut
855.4.SMILOW • yalecancercenter.org

Index

Made in the USA
Monee, IL
22 April 2022

95213320R00019